Medical Terminology

Medical Terminology Made Easy: Breakdown the Language of Medicine and Quickly Build Your Medical Vocabulary

Eva Regan

ISBN: 1532921519
ISBN-13: 978-1532921513

Contents

This book is not intended as a substitute for the medical advice of physicians. The reader should regularly consult a physician in matters relating to his/her health and particularly with respect to any symptoms that may require diagnosis or medical attention.

Section 1: Introduction

Medical terminology is the language that is used to describe everything from human anatomy and physiology, to clinical conditions, diagnoses, processes, and procedures. It is the language medical professionals use to effectively and efficiently communicate with one another in a science-based manner. It is used to wrap several words into one word, thereby making communication significantly more time-efficient. It therefore allows doctors, nurses, and other medical professionals to convey a lot of information in the most concise and precise way. With that said, having a sound understanding of medical terminology is a key skill that should be sharpened by every health care professional.

The good news is that you likely already have a good medical vocabulary! If you study or work in a medical setting, you already use medical words every day. Many medical terms such as arthritis, hepatitis, or leukemia are already commonly used in common language, whilst other medical words are more complicated. The aim of this guide is to help you become fluent and breakdown unknown and more complicated words and interpret their meanings.

In this book, you will find extensive alphabetical lists of root words, prefixes, and suffixes, explanations and examples, as well as the terms that are specific to parts of the body and body systems. We will also cover how to deconstruct a medical term and decipher its meaning, how to pluralize, and much more!

At the end of this guide, you'll be able to:

- Understand the logic of medical terminology and apply it to your profession.
- Build medical terms from scratch using prefixes, root words, combining forms, and suffixes that you have learned in this guide.
- Deconstruct complicated words and use the word elements to analyze and determine the meaning of the medical terms.
- Understand, spell, and write medical words. Use them to communicate and document any health care situation with accuracy and precision.
- Explain the meaning of medical terms to other people.

After all, medical terminology is just like a jigsaw puzzle! Through identifying and recognizing the root, the prefix, and the suffix of a term, you will be able to deconstruct and understand any medical term, and build a strong vocabulary.

Remember that mastering medical terminology is like mastering a language – it requires practice, hard work, and determination. But at the same time, it is also a lot of fun once you have mastered it and can put it into great use!

Best wishes,

Eva Regan

Section 2: Etymology

When dealing with medical terminology, it is important to remember that each word is 'organic' in the sense that you can trace it back to its specific meaning. Etymology is the study of the origin of the word. Etymology can be used to interpret acronyms, eponyms, and words with Greek or Latin origins. Acronyms are abbreviations or modern terms which are used to describe longer terms and phrases, and eponyms are words that are named after people.

Like with any other language, it is through breaking down a word into different 'parts' that you can gain an understanding of the meaning of the word. The different 'parts' which we will constantly refer back to in this book include the following:

- **Root Words:** The root word is the core meaning of the term and the foundations on which the medical term is built. It usually specifies the body part to which the word refers to. Both prefixes and suffixes must always be attached to a root word. A **combining vowel** is a vowel that connects a root word to another root word or a suffix. The vowel 'o' is the most common combining vowel. The vowels 'a', 'i', and 'u' are used less frequently. In the lists that are provided in the sections to follow, the combining vowel will always be given in brackets behind the root word. A

combining form is the combination of a root word and a combining vowel.

- **Prefixes:** Prefixes appear at the beginning of a word and usually supplies information as to the circumstance which surround the meaning of the word. They usually give you a hint as to what to expect from a word through indicating one or more of the following: how, how much, how many, why, where, when, the position, status, time, or direction.

- **Suffixes:** Suffixes appear at the end of a word. They usually inform you as to what is happening with a specific component or system of the body by indicating one of the following: a condition, disease, or procedure.

Every medical term will have a root word, some will have a prefix, some will have a suffix, and some will have both a suffix and a prefix. Each root word, prefix, and suffix has its very own specific meaning. Let's take the suffix '-ectomy' for example. Because '-ectomy' is a suffix, it is to be found at the end of a term. '-Ectomy' means "surgical removal of." With this in mind, we know that 'Tonsillectomy' refers to the surgical removal of the tonsils and that 'Appendectomy' describes the surgical removal of the appendix.

Essentially every medical word can be broken down into

roots, prefixes, and suffixes. Because the root is the main part of a word, there are significantly more root words than there are prefixes and suffixes. In the next chapter we have put together a list of the most important root words, the knowledge of which is central to mastering medical terminology!

Section 3: Deconstructing and Analyzing Medical Terminology

This section is split up into four parts. In the first part, you will learn how to break down medical terminology. You will then have the chance to break down words yourself and define their meaning accordingly. In the last two parts of this section, we will show you how to build medical vocabulary from scratch using the words that you have learned in the previous sections.

Before we dive into how to break down medical terminology, it is important to recall the elements that make up a medical term, which include the following:

- Prefix – the beginning of some words
- Root word(s)
- Combining vowel
- Combining form (= root word + combining vowel)
- Suffix – the end of some words

1. *Break it down in 3 Steps!*

Deconstructing medical terminology is easy and you can do so in three simple steps! When deconstructing medical terminology, the first rule is to **always** start at the end. That is with the suffix – identify the suffix and determine its meaning. The second step is to look at the beginning of the word, to recognize any prefix and determine its meaning. The final step is then to identify the root, its meaning, and assemble all the identified meanings.

Let's take the word 'Endocarditis' for example. Breaking it down into its individual components we have: ENDO – CARD – ITIS.

- We know that the suffix 'itis' stands for 'inflammation'
- We recognize that 'endo' is the prefix which stands for 'inside'
- Finally, 'card' is the root word for 'heart'

Assembling the three meanings: we therefore know that Endocarditis has a meaning of 'inflammation of the inside of the heart'!

Let's take another word: Hematology: HEMAT – O – LOGY.

- We know that the suffix 'logy' stands for 'study of'
- Hemat at the beginning of the sentence is not a prefix but rather a root words which means 'blood'

- O – the O in this case is the combining vowel which is often found in medical terms to ease pronunciation and to connect a root word and another root word or a root word in a suffix (note that it is never placed between a prefix and a root word). 'Hemato' is the combining form.

Putting the two meanings together ('study of' and 'blood'), we therefore know that Hematology means 'study of blood'.

The three simple steps to deconstruct a medical term are therefore as follows:

1. Identify the suffix at the end of the word and define its meaning.
2. Recognize any prefix/root word at the beginning of the word and and define its meaning.
3. Recognize the root/middle section and define its meaning.

Once deconstructed, assemble the meanings together to define the meaning of the word.

2. *Test Yourself: Deconstructing Medical Terms*

This part is designed to help you practice breaking down medical words. The answers are given at the end. Do not worry if you don't know the meaning of the different word parts yet, but rather focus on breaking the word down into its main components. Feel free to revisit this section once you have learned the root words, prefixes, and suffixes provided in the lists in *Sections 4, 5 and 6.*

Exercises:

Exercise 1: Arthroophthalmopathy

Exercise 2: Arthroscopy

Exercise 3: Cerebromalacia

Exercise 4: Costochondral

Exercise 5: Encephalomegaly

Exercise 6: Esophagogastroduodenoscopy

Exercise 7: Hemigastrectomy

Exercise 8: Leiomyosarcoma

Exercise 9: Pneumoconiosis

Exercise 10: Retrogastric

Answers:

Answer 1: '-pathy' stands for disease or condition + 'Arthr' means joint + 'ophthalmo' means eye = Arthroophthalmopathy which is a disease affecting the joints and the eyes. Notice here that even though the second root word starts with a vowel, a combining vowel is nevertheless required to connect one root word to another.

Answer 2: '-scopy' stands for 'visual examination of' + Arthro means joint = Arthroscopy is therefore the visual examination of a joint.

Answer 3: '-malacia' means softening + 'Cerebro' is related to the brain = Cerebromalacia which is the softening of the brain.

Answer 4: '-al' stands for pertaining to + 'Costo' means rib + 'chandro' means cartilage. Costochondral therefore means 'pertaining to the ribs and the cartilage.

Answer 5: '-megaly' means enlargement + Encephalo means brain = Encephalomegaly which is the enlargement of the brain.

Answer 6: '-scopy' stands for visual examination of + 'Esophago' means esophagus + 'gastro' means stomach + 'duodeno' means duodenum = Esophagogastroduodenoscopy which is the visual examination of the esophagus, the stomach, and the duodenum.

Answer 7: '-ectomy' stands for surgical removal of + 'hemi' means half + 'gastr' means stomach = Hemigastrectomy which is the surgical removal of half the stomach.

Answer 8: '-sarcoma' is a malignant tumor + 'Leio' stands for smooth' + 'myo' means muscle = Leiomyosarcoma which is a tumor of the smooth muscle.

Answer 9: '-sis' stands for condition + 'Pneumo' means lung

+ 'conio' stands for dust = Pneumoconiosis which is a lung condition caused by the inhalation of dust particles or matter.

Answer 10: '-ic' stands for pertaining to + 'Retro' is a prefix that means behind + 'gastr' means stomach = Retrogastric which therefore means pertaining to behind the stomach.

3. Building Medical Terms using 3 rules!

Medical words are made up of four types of word parts. We have already covered the three substantive word parts in *Section 2*.

1. Prefix
2. Root word
3. Combining Vowel
4. Suffix

By connecting various word parts, you can build thousands of words. There are three rules for building medical words using the elements above:

1. A prefix is always placed at the beginning of the word

2. A suffix is always placed at the end of the word
3. If there is more than one root word, a combining vowel is always needed to separate the root words even if the root word already begins with a vowel.

Always start with the root word and add a suffix (and/or/if required the prefix) and a combining vowel if necessary. Therefore, for example, if we wanted to build a medical word that means 'disease of the brain', we would start with the root word for brain which is 'encephal'. We also know that the suffix for disease is '-pathy'. To connect the two parts and to ease pronunciation, we will also add the combining vowel 'o'.

ENCEPHAL – O – PATHY = brain disease

Let's try something more complicated. Let's say we wanted to say that our client is suffering from an inflammation of the larynx, trachea, and the bronchus. We can express this using just one word! We would start with the three root words in this case:

- 'Laryng' for larynx,
- 'Trache' for trachea, and
- 'Bronch' for bronchus.

We know that the '-itis' is the suffix that stands for inflammation. We have also learned in the previous section that a combining vowel is always needed to connect one root word to another. Equipped with this knowledge, we therefore know that the medical term we are after must therefore be 'laryngotracheobronchitis':

LARYNG – O – TRACHE – O – BRONCH – IT IS = inflammation of the larynx, trachea, and bronchus

4. *Test Yourself: Building Medical Terms*

This part is designed to help you practice building medical terms. You may or may not already know the word parts necessary to build these terms. Do not worry if you don't know them because you will have an opportunity to learn about them later. In the next three sections, you are provided with alphabetical listings of word parts. If you do not feel equipped for this exercise yet, I would suggest going through the lists of word parts once or twice and then revisit these exercises once you feel prepared.

Exercises

Exercise 1: Condition or disease affecting the bones and joints

Exercise 2: Excessive amount of cholesterol in the blood

Exercise 3: Inflammation around a nerve

Exercise 4: Incision into the salivary gland to remove a stone

Exercise 5: Insufficient or low amount of sugar in the blood

Exercise 6: An X-ray record of the uterus and the Fallopian tube

Exercise 7: Stomach ache

Exercise 8: Surgical fixation of the urethra to a nearby tissue

Exercise 9: Enlargement of the internal organs

Exercise 10: The branch of medicine that deals with disorders of the stomach and the intestines

Answers

Answer 1: Because we have two root words here, we know that we will need a combining vowel to connect the two. 'Oste' means bones + 'arthr' means bones + '-pathy' is the suffix pertaining to a condition or disease = Osteoarthropathy (OSTE – O – ARTHR – O PATHY). The second vowel is necessary here to ease pronunciation.

Answer 2: '-emia' is the suffix pertaining to blood condition + 'cholesterol' is the root word + 'hyper-' is the prefix which means excessive or above normal = Hypercholesterolemia (HYPER – CHOLESTEROL – EMIA).

Answer 3: '-itis' is the suffix that stands for inflammation + 'neur' means nerve + 'peri-' is the prefix that stands for around = Perineuritis (PERI – NEUR – ITIS).

Answer 4: '-otomy' is the suffix that stands for surgical incision into + 'sial' means salivary gland + 'lith' means stone or calculus = Sialolithotomy (SIAL – O – LITH – OTOMY).

Answer 5: '-emia' is the suffix pertaining to blood condition + 'glyc' means sugar + 'hypo-' is the prefix that stands for insufficient or below normal = Hypoglycemia (HYPO – GLYC – EMIA).

Answer 6: '-gram' is the suffix that stands for record + 'hyster' means uterus + 'salping' means Fallopian tube = Hysterosalpingogram (HYSTER – O – SALPING – GRAM). The first combining vowel is always required here because it is necessary to connect two root words (even if one starts with a vowel) and the second combining vowel is required to ease pronunciation.

Answer 7: '-dynia' is the suffix for ache or pain + 'gastr' means stomach = Gastrodynia (GASTR – O – DYNIA).

Answer 8: '-pexy' is the suffix for surgical fixation + 'urethr' is the root word that means urethra = Urethropexy (URETHR – O – PEXY).

Answer 9: '-megaly' is the suffix for enlargement + 'viscer' is the root word for viscera (organs) = Visceromegaly (VISCER – O – MEGALY).

Answer 10: '-ology' is the suffix that stands for 'the study of' + 'gastr' means stomach + 'enter' means intestines = Gastroenterology (GASTR – O – ENTER – OLOGY).

Section 4: Know Your Root Words!

Below are the most important and most common root words that can appear before any suffix an after any prefix. Root words usually derive from the Latin or Greek language and are divided into two main categories. **Exterior root words** are word components that describe everything on the exterior of the body. **Interior root words** are word components that describe everything inside the body.

1. Exterior Root Words

'A' Exterior Root Word = Meaning

Acr(o) = Extremities, topmost

Amb(i) = Both sides, double

Anter(o) = Front

Aut(o) = Self

Axill(o) = Axilla, armpit

'B' Exterior Root Word = Meaning

Blephar(o) = Eyelid, eyelash

Brachi(o) = Arm

Bucc(o) = Cheek (face)

An example being **Blepharo**plasty (the surgical repair of the eyelids).

'C' Exterior Root Word = Meaning

Canth(o) = Angle formed where the eyelids meet

Capit(o) = Head

Cephal(o) = Head

Carp(o) = Wrist

Caud(o) = Tail, downward

Cervic(o) = Neck, cervix

Cheil(o), Chil(o) = Lip

Cheir(o), Chir(o) = Hand

Cili(o) = Eyelash, eyelid

Cor(e), Cor(o) = Pupil

Crani(o) = Skull

Cubit(o) = Elbow

Examples include:

- **Cephalo**centesis (the surgical puncture of the skull),
- **Cervico**dynia (neck pain),

- **Cheilo**phagia (biting of the lip), and
- **Cheiro**megaly (enlargement of the hand).

'D' Exterior Root Word = Meaning

Dactyl(o) = Fingers or toes

Derm(a/o), Dermat(o) = Skin

Dors(i), Dors(o) = Back, posterior

Examples include:

- **Derma**tome (the instrument used for cutting thin skin slices), and
- **Dors**algia (back pain).

'F' Exterior Root Word = Meaning

Faci(o) = Face

'G' Exterior Root Word = Meaning

Gingiv(o) = Gums (mouth)

Gloss(o) = Tongue

Gnath(o) = Jaws

An example being **Gingiv**itis (inflammation of the gums).

'I' Exterior Root Word = Meaning

Inguin(o) = Groin

Irid(o) = Iris (eye)

'L' Exterior Root Word = Meaning

Labi(o) = Lips

Lapar(o) = Abdomen, flank

Later(o) = Side

Lingu(o) = Tongue

Examples being:

- **Laparo**scopy (the visual examination of the abdomen), and
- Sub**lingu**al (under or below the tongue).

'M' Exterior Root Word = Meaning

Mamm(a/o) = Breast

Mast(o) = Breast

Examples include:

- **Mammo**plasty (the surgical repair of the breast(s)), and
- **Mast**ectomy (the surgical removal of the breast(s)).

'N' Exterior Root Word = Meaning

Nas(o) = Nose

'O' Exterior Root Word = Meaning

Occipit(o) = Back of the head

Ocul(o) = Eye

Odont(o) = Teeth

Omphal(o) = Umbilicus

Onych(o) = Nails

Ophtalm(o), ocul(o) = Eyes

Optic(o), opt(o) = Sight, seeing

Or(o) = Mouth

Ot(o) = Ear

Examples include:

- **Odont**algia (toothache),
- **Onycho**malacia (softening of the nails),
- **Oro**lingual (pertaining to the mouth), and

- **Oto**dynia (earache).

'P' Exterior Root Word = Meaning

Papill(o) = Nipple

Pelv(i/o) = Pelvis

Phall(o) = Hair

Pil(o) = Foot

Pod(o) = Foot

Examples include:

- **Pelvi**metry (measurement of the pelvis), and
- **Pod**arthritis (inflammation fo the joints of the foot).

'R' Exterior Root Word = Meaning

Rhin(o) = Nose

Examples include:

- **Rhino**plasty (the surgical repair of the nose), and
- **Rhino**rrhea (the discharge or flow of mucus from the nose).

'S' Exterior Root Word = Meaning

Somat(o) = Body

Steth(o) = Chest

Stomat(o) = Mouth

An example being **Stomat**itis (the inflammation of the inner lining of the mouth).

'T' Exterior Root Word = Meaning

Tal(o) = Ankle

Tars(o) = Foot

Thorac(o) = Chest, thorax

Trachel(o) = Neck, neckline

Trich(i/o) = Hair, hair-like structure

Examples include:

- **Thorac**entesis (the surgical puncture into the chest cavity), and
- **Thorac**otomy (the surgical incision into the chest cavity).

'V' Exterior Root Word = Meaning

Ventr(i/o) = Front of the body

2. *Interior Root Words*

'A' Interior Root Word = Meaning

Abdomin(o) = Abdomen

Acanth(o) = Spiny, thorny

Acetabul(o) = Acetabulum

Acromi(o) = Acromium

Aden(o) = Gland

Adip(o) = Fat, fatty tissue

Adren(o) = Adrenal gland

Alveoli(o) = Air sac

Angi(o) = Blood vessel

An(o) = Anus

Aort(o) = Aorta

Arteri(o), Arter(o) = Artery

Arteriol(o) = Arteriole

Aspir(o) = Breathing in

Ather(o) = Fatty deposit

Athr(o), Articul(o) = Joint

Atri(o) = Atrium

Audi(o), Aur(i) = Hearing

Examples include:

- **Abdomino**plasty (the surgical repair of the abdomen),
- **Adeno**megaly (enlargement of a gland),
- Angio**plasty** (the surgical repaid of a vessel),
- Arterio**plasty** (the surgical repair of an artery),
- Arthro**plasty** (the surgical repair of a joint),
- **Atrio**megaly (enlargement of an atrium of the heart), and
- **Audio**metry (the measurement of hearing).

'B' Interior Root Word = Meaning

Balan(o) = Glans penis, glans clitoris

Bio- = Life

Bronch(i/o) = Bronchus (plural bronchi)

Bronchiol(i/o) = Bronchiole

Examples include:

- **Bio**logy (the study of life, the study of living organisms),
- **Bronchi**tis (inflammation of the bronchi), and

- **Broncho**scopy (the visual examination of the bronchi.

'C' Interior Root Word = Meaning

Carcin(o) = Cancer

Cardi(o) = Heart

Cellul(o) = Cell

Cerebell(o) = Cerebellum

Cerebr(i/o) = Cerebrum

Cholangi(o) = Bile duct

Chol(e) = Bile

Cholecyst(o) = Gallbladder

Choledoch(o) = Common bile duct

Chondr(i/o) = Cartrilage

Chrom(o), Chromat(o) = Color

Col(o), Colon(o) = Colon

Colp(o) = Vagina

Cost(o) = Rib

Cry(o) = Cold

Crypt(o) = Hidden

Cutane(o) = Skin

Cyan(o) = Blue

Cysti, Cyst(o) = Bladder, cyst

Cyt(o) = Cell

Examples include:

- **Carcino**gen (a cancer-producing substance),
- **Cardi**ac (pertaining to the heart),
- **Cardi**tis (inflammation of the heart),
- **Cryo**biology (the branch of biology that deals with the effects of low temperatures),
- **Cysto**gram (a radiograph of the bladder),
- **Cyano**sis (bluish discoloration of the skin), and
- **Cyt**ology (the study of cells).

'D' Interior Root Word = Meaning

Dipl(o) = Twice, double

Duoden(o) = Duodenum

Examples include:

- **Diplo**pia (condition of double vision), and
- **Duoden**ectomy (surgical removal of the duodenum).

'E' Interior Root Word = Meaning

Encephal(o) = Brain

Enter(o) = Intestine

Episi(o) = Vulva

Erythr(o) = Red

Esophag(o) = Esophagus

Examples include:

- **Encephalo**pathy (a disease or disorder of the brain),
- **Episi**otomy (the surgical cutting of the vulva),
- **Eryth**ema (reddening of the skin), and
- **Esophago**gastroduodenoscopy or EDG (visual examination of the esophagus, the duodenum and the stomach).

'F' Interior Root Word = Meaning

Fibr(o) = Fibers

'G' Interior Root Word = Meaning

Galact(o) = Milk

Gastr(o) = Stomach

Glyc(o) = Sugar

Gynec(o) = Female

Examples include:

- **Galacto**rrhea (flow of milk when nursing),
- **Gastro**dynia (stomach ache), and
- **Glyco**suria (presence of sugar in the urine).

'H' Interior Root Word = Meaning

Hemat(o), Hem(o) = Blood

Hepat(o), Hepatic(o) = Liver

Heter(o) = Different, other

Hidr(o) = Sweat

Hist(o), Histi(o) = Tissue

Hom(o), Home(o) = Alike, same

Hydr(o) = Water

Hyster(o) = Uterus

Examples include:

- **Hemat**emesis (vomiting of blood),
- **Hemato**cyte (blood cell),
- **Hepato**megaly (enlargement of the liver),
- **Histo**logy (the study of tissue),
- **Hydro**penia (deficiency of water in the body), and
- **Hyster**ectomy (surgical removal of the uterus).

'I' Interior Root Word = Meaning

Ile(o) = Ileum (intestine)

Ili(o) = Ilium (pelvic bone)

Intestin(o) = Intestine

Examples include:

- **Ileo**stomy (the artificial or surgical opening into the ileum), and
- **Illio**inguinal (pertaining to the ilium).

'J' Interior Root Word = Meaning

Jejun(o) = Jejunum

Examples include:

- **Jejun**itis (inflammation of the jejunum), and
- **Jejuno**stomy (surgical or artificial opening into the jejunum).

'K' Interior Root Word = Meaning

Kerat(o) = Cornea (eye or skin)

'L' Interior Root Word = Meaning

Latr(o) = Treatment

Lacrima = Tears

Laryng(o) = Larynx

Leuk(o) = White

Lipid(o) = Fat

Lith(o) = Stone (gallbladder or kidney)

Lymph(o) = Lymph

Examples include:

- **Lacrima**tory (causing a flow of tears),
- **Laryng**itis (inflammation of the larynx),
- **Leuko**cyte (white blood cell), and
- **Litho**tripsy (the crushing of a stone or calculus).

'M' Interior Root Word = Meaning

Melan(o) = Black

Men(o) = Menstruation, menses

Mening(o) = Meninges

Metr(a/o) = Uterus

My(o) = Muscle

Myel(o) = Bonne marrow, spinal cord

Myring(o) = Eardrum

Examples include:

- **Melano**ma (tumor or growth that is black-colored),
- **Myelo**gram (recording of the spinal cord), and
- **Myo**sitis (inflammation of the muscle).

'N' Interior Root Word = Meaning

Nat(o) = Birth

Necr(o) = Death

Nephr(o) = Kidney

Neur(o) = Nerve

Examples include:

- **Necro**sis (condition of cell death),
- **Nephro**lithiasis (condition of kidney stones),
- **Neuro**logist (a physician who treats and studies conditions relating to the nervous system), and
- Pre**natal**/post**natal** (before/after birth).

'O' Interior Root Word = Meaning

Oophor(o) = Ovary

Orchid(o), Orchi(o) = Testis

Oss(i/eo), Ost(e/eo) = Bone

Examples include:

- **Oophp**rectomy (the surgical removal of an ovary), and
- **Orchi**algia (pain in the testicle).

'P' Interior Root Word = Meaning

Palat(o) = Roof of the mouth

Path(o) = Disease

Peritone(o) = Peritoneum

Pharmac(o) = Drug

Pharyng(o) = Pharynx

Phleb(o) = Vein

Phren(o) = Diaphragm

Pleur(o) = Ribs, pleura

Pneum(a/o/ato/ono) = Lungs

Pulmon(o) = Lungs

Poli(o) = Grey color

Proct(o) = Anus, rectum

Py(o) = Pus

Pyel(o) = Pelvis (kidney)

Examples include:

- **Patho**logy (branch of medicine that covers the study of diseases),
- **Peritone**al (pertaining to the peritoneum),
- **Pharyng**itis (inflammation of the pharynx),
- **Pneumo**coniosis (condition of abnormal deposits of matter in the lungs), and
- **Pyelo**lithotomy (removal of a stone from the pelvis).

'R' Interior Root Word = Meaning

Rect(o) = Rectum

Ren(i/o) = Kidney

An example being **Recto**sigmoid (pertaining to the rectum and the sigmoid).

'S' Interior Root Word = Meaning

Sacr(o) = Sacrum

Salping(o) = Fallopian tube

Sarc(o) = Flesh

Scapul(o) = Scapula

Sept(o) = Infection

Splen(o) = Spleen

Spondyl(o) = Vertebra

Stern(o) = Sternum

Examples include:

- **Salping**ectomy (surgical removal of the fallopian tube),
- **Sarco**id (resembling flesh),
- **Sept**icemia (blood poisoning, presence of toxins and pathogenic organisms in the blood), and
- **Spleno**megaly (enlargement of the spleen).

'T' Interior Root Word = Meaning

Ten(o), Tend(o), Tendin(o) = Tendon

Testicul(o) = Testis

Therm(o) = Heat

Thorac(o) = Chest

Thym(o) = Thymus

Thyr(o), Thyroid(o) = Thyroid gland

Tonsill(o) = Tonsils

Trache(o) = Trachea

Tympan(o) = Eardrum

Examples include:

- **Tendin**itis or **Tendo**nitis (inflammation of a tendon),
- **Testicul**ar (pertaining to the testicles),
- **Thoraco**tomy (incision into the cavity of the chest), and
- **Tonsill**ectomy (surgical removal of the tonsils).

'U' Interior Root Word = Meaning

Ur(e/o/ea/eo), Urin(o) = Urine

Ureter(o) = Ureter

Urethr(o) = Urethra

Uter(o) = Uterus

Examples include:

- **Uretero**lith (stone or calculus in the ureter),
- **Urethro**rrhea (abnormal or excessive discharge from the urethra), and
- **Urethro**pexy (surgical fixation of the urethra).

'V' Interior Root Word = Meaning

Vas(o) = Vas deferens

Vas(o), Ven(i/o) = Vein

Vesic(o) = Bladder

Viscer(o) = Viscera (internal organs)

Examples include:

- **Vas**ectomy (surgical removal of a portion of the vas deferens), and
- **Viscer**omegaly or Organomegaly (enlargement of the viscera, enlargement of the internal organs).

'X' Interior Root Word = Meaning

Xanth(o) = Yellowness

Xer(o) = Dry

Although this list may appear discouraging, learning and being able to recognize these root words will really have a huge impact on your understanding of medical terminology and on your career altogether!

In the next section, we will be covering prefixes and suffixes and how they can help you decipher medical terms.

3. *Directional Root Words*

Directional root words are directional words that refer to a certain part or area of the body.

Directional Root Word = Meaning

Anter(o) = Front

Caud(o) = Tail, downward
Cephal(o) = Head, upward
Dist(o) = Away from

Dors(o) = Back

Infer(o) = Below

Later(o) = Side

Medi(o) = Middle

Poster(o) = Back, behind

Proxim(o) = Near (proximate)

Super(o) = Above

Ventr(o) = Front, belly

In summary therefore:

- **Anter**ior and **ventr**al are used when referring to the front of the body.
- **Poster**ior and **dors**al are used when referring to the back of the body.
- **Cephal**ad and **super**ior are used when referring to 'above the waistline.'
- **Caud**al and **infer**ior are used when referring to 'below the waistline.'
- **Later**al is used when referring to the sides of the body.
- **Medi**al is used when referring to the middle of the body.

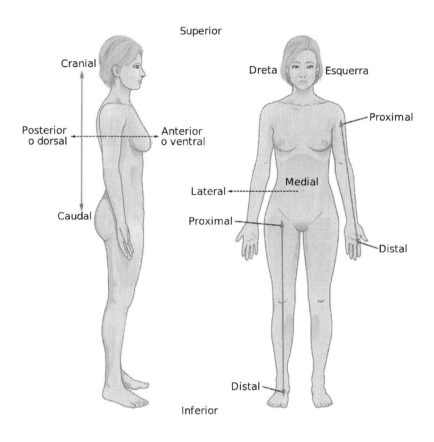

Section 5: Prefixes

We have already discussed the role of prefixes in *Section 2.* In this section, we will provide a brief recap as well as a list of the most common and most important prefixes and relevant examples.

1. *The Most Important Prefixes*

Prefixes, which are always at the beginning of a word, are designed to inform you about the circumstances which surround the word. Below is a list of the most important prefixes in medical terminology, a lot of which you would already be familiar with!

Prefix = Meaning

A-, an- = Without, not, lack of

Ab- = Away from, take away

Ad- = Toward, near

Ambi-, ambo- = Both

Amphi- = Double, both sides

Ana-, ante- = Before, forward, in front of

Anti- = Against, opposing

Ap-, apo- = Separated, derived from

Aut-, auto- = Self, by yourself

Examples include:

- **A**menorrhea (the absence/lack of a period or menstruation),
- **An**ovulatory (a menstrual cycle without ovulation),
- **Ab**duction (the movement of a body part or limb away from the midline of the body),
- **Ad**duction (the movement of a body part toward the body's midline), and
- **Anti-**inflammatory (a drug or agent which opposed inflammation in the body).

Bi- = Two, double, both, twice
Brady- = Slow

Brachy = Short

Examples include:

- **Bi**lateral (affecting/relating to both sides),
- **Brady**cardia (slow heart rate), and
- **Brady**arrhythmia (a slow and irregular heartbeat).

Cata- = Lower, down, against

Circum- = Around

Co-, con-, com-, cor- = With, together

Contra- = Against, opposed to

Examples include:

- **Circum**ferential (around the outside), and
- **Contra**indication (to be avoided: some medications are contraindicated in the presence of other medications).

De- = Down, from

Di- = Two, twice

Dia- = Through, between, across, apart

Dis- = Apart from, free from

Dys- = Difficult, bad, painful

Examples include:

- **Dys**functional (difficult or painful), and
- **Dis**section (to cut or slice something into two parts).

E-, ec-, ex- = From, away from, out of

Ect-, exo-, ecto- = Outside, outer, on

Em-, en- = In

End-, endo-, ent-, ento- = Within, inner

Epi-, ep- = Upon, over, on

Eu- = Normal

Extra-, extro- = Outside of, beyond, outward

Examples include:

- **Exo**cervix (the protective mucous membrane one the outside of the cervix), and
- **Endo**cervix (the inner part of the cervix).

Hemi-, semi- = Half, half of

Hyper-, Ultra- = Excessive, beyond, above

Hyp-, Hypo- = Deficient, beneath, below

Examples include:

- **Hyper**tension (excessive or high or above normal blood pressure),
- **Hyper**emesis (excessive vomiting), and
- **Hypo**tensive (low or below normal blood pressure).

Im-, in- = Into, in, within

Infra- = Below, beneath

Inter- = Between

Intra- = Within, inside

Intro- = Within, into

Examples include:

- **Infra**umbilical (below or beneath the umbilicus),
- **Intra**uterine device (a contraceptive device that is used inside or within the uterus),
- **Intra**venous (injection within a vein, within a vein), and
- **Intra**muscular (injection into a muscle, not between a muscle).

Macro- = Large

Micro-, micr- = Small, tiny

Mal- = Bad

Mes-, meso- = Middle

Meta- = Beyond, changing
Mono-, uni- = One

Mult-, multi- = Multiple

Examples include:

- **Macro**scopic (large enough to be seen with the natural eye),
- **Micro**scopic (very small, only visible with a microscope),

- **Multi**loculated (a tumor or cyst with multiple cavities), and
- **Multi**parous (having borne more than one child).

Neo- = New, recent

Examples include:

- **Neo**plasia (the condition of new or recent growth, usually pertaining to cells), and
- **Neo**plasm (new or recent growth, e.g. of a tumor).

Oligo-, oil- = Scanty

Examples include:

- **Olig**luria (scanty or inadequate amount of urine production), and
- **Oligo**menorrhea (scanty period, scanty menstrual flow).

Pan- = All

Para- = Beyond, beside, after

Per- = Through

Peri- = Around

Poly- = Excessive, many

Post- = After, following, behind

Pre-, pro- = Before, preceding, in front of

Presby- = Old age

Pseudo: = False

Examples include:

- **Para**ovarian (beside the ovary),
- **Peri**cardial (around the heart),
- **Peri**urethral (around the opening of the urethra),
- **Peri**operative (the period of time around (the time of) surgery),
- **Poly**dipsia (excessive thirst),
- **Poly**uria (excessive amount of urine production),
- **Post**natal (after giving birth)
- **Pre**natal (before giving birth),
- **Post**operative (the period of time after surgery),
- **Pre**operative (the period of time before surgery),
- **Pre**menstrual (the period of time before the menstrual period begins),
- **Pseudo**cyst (a structure that resembles a cyst), and
- **Pseudo**pregnancy (a false pregnancy).

Quadri- = Four

Re- = Backward, again

Retro- = Behind, backward

Semi- = Half

Sub- = Under, beneath

Super-, supra- = Superior, excessive, above

Sym-, syn- = With, together

Examples include:

- **Sub**costal (under or beneath the ribs), and
- **Sub**umbilical (the area underneath or beneath the umbilicus).

Tachy- = Fast

Trans- = Through, across

Tri- = Three

Examples include:

- **Tachy**cardia (a rapid or fast heart rate), and
- **Tachy**arrhythmia (a rapid or fast arrhythmia).

Ultra- = Excessive, beyond

2. *Prefixes and Medical Antonyms*

Prefix = Meaning

Ab- = Abduction, away from

Ad- = Adduction, toward

Anterior- = Front

Posterior- = Back

Bio- = Life

Necro- = Death

Brady- = Slow

Tachy- = Fast

Cephalo- = Upward (head)

Caudo- = Downward (tail)

Endo- = Inside, within

Exo- = Outside

Eu- = Well, normal

Dys- = Unwell, difficult

Hyper- = Excessive, above

Hpo- = Deficient, below

Leuko- = White

Melano- = Black

Macro- = Large

Micro- = mall

Pre- = Before, in front of

Post- = After, behind

Proximal- = Near (in terms of proximity)

Distal- = Away from (in terms of distance)

There are some prefixes above that look similar but do in fact mean the opposite. These are the 'faux-amis' among the prefixes. Note these down and watch out for them!

3. *Prefixes and Medical Synonyms*

There are some prefixes which may look entirely different but do in fact share the same meaning. The most common among this group include the following:

- *Ante-*, *pro-* and *pre-* all mean 'before'
- *Anti-* and *contra-* both mean 'against'
- *Dys-* and *mal-* both mean 'painful' or 'bad'
- *Hyper-*, *supra-* and *epi-* all mean 'above'
- *Hypo-*, *sub-* and *infra-* all mean 'below'
- *Intra-* and *endo-* both mean 'within'

4. *Prefixes for Positions and Directions*

In the medical or surgical setting, you will often encounter terms that identify a specific location in the body. Sometimes you will also be required to use appropriate language to describe body positions that indicate how the patient should be placed during procedures, or the necessary direction of any movement and part of the body. In this section, we will cover the main prefixes that relating to position and direction that you will need to successfully navigate and guide your patients.

Prefix = Meaning

Ab- = Away from

Ad- = Toward

Circum- = Around

Contra- = Opposition, against

De- = Down, away from

Ecto-, Exo- = Outside

Endo- = Within

Epi- = Upon, over

Extra- = Outside

Infra- (sub) = Below, under

Intra- = Inside

Ipsi- (iso) = Same (equal)

Ir- = Into, toward

Meso- = Middle

Meta- (supra) = Beyond, over, after

Para- = Near, beside

Peri- = Around, surrounding

Retro- = Behind, backward

Sub- = Under, rear,

Trans- = Across, through

Examples include:

- **Exo**genous (caused by outside factors),
- **Endo**crine (pertaining to internal secretions),
- **Epi**gastric (the upper and middle region of the abdomen),
- **Infra**sternal (below or under the sternum),
- **Meta**stasis (the transfer of a disease from one organ to body part to another),
- **Peri**odontal (around the tooth), and
- **Retro**peritoneal (behind the peritoneum).

5. _Prefixes for Numbers and Measurements_

In this section we will cover all the prefixes relating to numbers as well as those relating to standard measurement.

Prefixes for number:

Prefix = Meaning

Uni-, Mono- = One, e.g. Unilateral

Bi-, Diplo- = Two, double, e.g. Bilateral

Gemin- = Double, pair, e.g. Gemini

Tri- = Three, e.g. Tricuspid

Quadri- = Four, e.g. Quadriplegic

Tetra- = Five, e.g. Quintipara

Sexti- = Six, e.g. Sextuplet

Septi- = Seven, e.g. Septuplet

Octa-, Octo- = Eight, e.g. Octahedron

Nona- = Nine, e.g. Nonan

Deca- = Ten, e.g. Decagram

Multi- = Many, multiple, e.g. Multicellular

Primi- = First, e.g. Primigravida

Semi-, Hemi- = Half, e.g. Semicircular

Ambi- = Both, both sides, e.g. Ambidextrous

Null- = None, e.g. Nullipara

Pan- = All, e.g. Pancytopenia

Prefixes for measurements:

Prefix = Numerical = Meaning

yotta- (Y-) = 10^{24} = 1 septillion

zetta- (Z-) = 10^{21} = 1 sextillion

exa- (E-) = 10^{18} = 1 quintillion

peta- (P-) = 10^{15} = 1 quadrillion

tera- (T-) = 10^{12} = 1 trillion

giga- (G-) = 10^9 = 1 billion

mega- (M-) = 10^6 = 1 million

kilo- (k-) = 10^3 = 1 thousand

hecto- (h-) = 10^2 = 1 hundred

deca- (da-) = 10 = Ten

deci- (d-) = 10^{-1} = 1 tenth

centi- (c-) = 10^{-2} = 1 hundredth

milli- (m-) = 10^{-3} = 1 thousandth

micro- (μ-) = 10^{-6} = 1 millionth

nano- (n-) = 10^{-9} = 1 billionth

pico- (p-) = 10^{-12} = 1 trillionth

femto- (f-) = 10^{-15} = 1 quadrillionth

atto- (a-) = 10^{-18} = 1 quintillionth

zepto- (z-) = 10^{-21} = 1 sextillionth

yocto- (y-) = 10^{-24} = 1 septillionth

Section 6: Suffixes

Suffixes, always at the end of a word, inform you what is being done with a specific body system or part. The suffix indicates a condition, disease, or procedure.

1. *The Most Important Suffixes*

Suffix = Meaning

-ac, -al, -ic, -ous, -tic = Pertaining to, related to

-algia, -dynia = Discomfort, pain

-arche = Beginning

-ate, -ize = Subject to

An example is My**algia** (muscle pain).

-cele = Protrusion (hernia)

-cidal, -cide = Something which kills or destroys

-cle, -cule, -ule, -ulus = Small

-cyte(s) = Cell(s)

Examples include:

- Erythro**cytes** (red blood cells) and
- Leuko**cytes** (white blood cells).

-desis = Surgical binding or fusion

-dynia = Pain

An example is Gastro**dynia** (stomach pain or discomfort).

-ectasis, -ectasia = Stretching, dilatation

-emesis = Vomit

-emia = Pertaining to blood or a blood condition

-ent, -er, -ist = Person

-esis, -iasis = Condition

Examples include:

- An**emia** (low or below normal hemoglobin in blood),
- Hyper**emesis** (excessive vomiting), and
- Leuk**emia** (blood condition related to white blood cells).

-form, -oid = Resembling, looking or shaped like

-genesis = Beginning of, origin of

-genic = Produced by

-graph = Instrument used to record something

-ism = Condition, theory

-itis = Inflammation

-lysis = Breakdown, destruction, separation

Examples include:

- Tonsill**itis** (inflammation of the tonsils),
- Bronch**itis** (inflammation of the bronchi), and
- Arthr**itis** (inflammation of the joint).

-malacia = Softening

-megaly = Enlargement

-meter = Instrument used to measure something
-metry = Process of measuring something

Examples include:

- Cardio**megaly** (enlargement of the heart),
- Hepato**megaly** (enlargement pf the liver),
- Spleno**megaly** (enlargement of the spleen), and
- Hepatospleno**megaly** (enlargement of the liver and the spleen).

-ologist = Specialist

-ology = Study

-oma = Tumor, growth

-opsy = To view

-osis = Process, condition

Examples include:

- Carcin**oma** (cancerous or malignant tumor),
- Nephr**osis** (a kidney condition),
- Leiomy**oma** (non-cancerous or benign tumor that arises from the smooth muscle – also called fibroid tumor),
- Melan**oma** (tumor of the melanocytic system of the skin (of melanin-forming cells) which is associated with skin cancer), and
- Psych**ologist** (psychology specialist).

-pathy = Disease

-penia = Deficiency, lack of

-pexy, -pexis = Surgical fixation

-phagia, -phagy = To eat

-phobia = Intolerance, morbid fear
-plasia = Formation, development

-plegia = Paralysis

-pnea = Breathing

-poiesis, poietic = The production or manufacturing of something

-ptosis = Downward displacement, dropping

Examples include:

- Abdomino**plasty** (plastic surgery of the abdomen),
- Acro**phobia** (fear of heights),
- A**pnea** (the condition of not breathing),
- Cardiomypo**pathy** (chronic disease of the heart muscle),
- Cardio**pathy** (heart disease),
- Claustro**phobia** (fear of small or enclosed spaces),
- Dys**pnea** (pain or difficult breathing),
- Hemi**plegia** (the paralysis of one side of the body),
- Neuro**pathy** (disease of one or more peripheral nerves, disease involving the nervous system),
- Ortho**pnea** (inability to breathe properly),
- Osteo**pathy** (disease involving the bone),
- Osteo**penia** (deficiency in bone mass),

- Photo**phobia** (visual intolerance of light),
- Quadri**plegia** (paralysis of all four quadrants of the body),
- Rhino**plasty** (nose job), and
- Urethro**pexy** (surgical fixation of the trachea).

-rrhage, -rrhagia = Excessive discharge or flow

-rrhaphy = Fixation, suturing in place

-rrhea = Discharge or flow

-rrhexis = Breaking away, rupture

Examples include:

- Dia**rrhea** (flow or discharge of watery or loose stools),
- Hemo**rrhage** (excessive flow of blood),
- Meno**rrhea** (a heavy or excessive menstrual period),
- Myo**rraphy** (suture of fixation of the muscle), and
- Myo**rrhexis** (ruptured muscle).

-sclerosis = Hardening

-spasm = Involuntary, sudden

-stasis = Stopping, to stop

-tome = Instrument

-tripsy = Crushing

-trophic, -trophy = Development, growth

2. <u>Suffixes Pertaining to Surgical and Diagnostic Procedures</u>

The list of suffixes that pertain to medical procedures is relatively short. However, you will repeatedly come across these in the medical setting, therefore it is crucial that you become familiar with the suffixes listed below.

Suffix = Meaning

-centesis = A surgical puncture to aspirate or withdraw fluid

An example being Abdominocentesis (the surgical puncture of the abdominal cavity).

-clasis = Breaking, to break

Examples include Alveoloclasis (the breaking of the

alveolus) and Cranioclasis (the crushing or breaking of the fetal head during a difficult delivery).

-desis = Binding, fixation, fusion of two parts

Examples include Fasciodesis (the surgical binding of a fascia to another fascia or a tendon) and Tenodesis (the stabilization of a joint, the suture of the end of a tendon to a bone).

-ectomy = 'Surgical removal of'

Examples include Appendectomy (the surgical removal of the appendix), Oophorectomy (the surgical removal of an ovary), Prostatectomy (the surgical removal of the prostate), Salpingectomy (the surgical removal of the fallopian tube), and Salpingo-oophorectomy or Oophorosalpingectomy (the surgical removal of a tube and an ovary),

-otomy = Surgical incision, cutting into

Examples include Colotomy (the surgical cutting into the colon), Laparotomy (surgical cutting into the abdomen), and Tracheotomy (surgical cutting into the trachea).

-ostomy, -stomy = Surgical creation of an artificial opening

Examples include Colostomy (the artificial opening/surgical creation of an opening in the colon), Ileostomy (the artificial opening of the ileum), and Tracheostomy (artificial opening into the trachea).

-plasty = Surgical repair

Examples include Abdominoplasty (the surgical repair of the abdomen) and Mammoplasty (the surgical repair of the breasts).

-scope = Instrument used visually examine something

Examples include Bronchoscope (the instrument that is used to examine the bronchus) and Endoscope (the instrument that is used for international visual examination).

-scopy = Process of visual examination

Examples include Bronchoscopy (the visual examination of the bronchus using a bronchoscope) and Endoscopy (the visual examination using an endoscope).

-gram = Resulting record or picture, written record

Examples include the Cardiogram (the film that is produced during cardiography), Mammogram (the record that results from mammography), and Salpingogram (the record that results from salpingography).

-graphy = The process of recording a record or picture

Examples include Cardiography (the process of recording the activity of the heart), Mammography (the process of examining the breast), and Salpingography (the process of examining the fallopian tube.

-opsy = Medical examination or inspection

Examples include Autopsy (a postmortem examination) and Biopsy (a medical examination of tissue which is removed forma living organism in order to disover the cause or extent of a disease).

-pexy = Surgical fixation

Examples include Cystopexy (the surgical attachment of the urinary bladder or the gallbladder to the abdominal wall or another supporting structure) and Hysteropexy (the surgical fixation of an abnormally movable or misplaced uterus).

-pheresis = Removal, to remove

An example being Apheresis (procedure by which blood is withdrawn form a donor).

-rrhapy = Strengthen, to strengthen (usually with suture)

Examples include Colporrhapy (surgical procedure to suture the vaginal wall) and Hymenorraphy (the surgical restoration and strengthening of the hymen).

-tripsy = Crushing

An example being Lithotripsy (the medical procedure by which a kidney stone or another calculus is broken down into small pieces using ultrasound shock waves).

3. _Suffixes Pertaining to Pathological Conditions_

Suffix = Meaning

-algia, -dynia = Ache, pain

-asthenia = Weakness

-betes = To go

-cele = Tumor, hernia, cavity, swelling

-derma = Skin

-ectasis = Dilation, expansion

-edema = Swelling

-emesis = Vomiting

-itis = Inflammation

-kinesis = Pertaining to motion

-lepsy = Seizure

-malacia = Softening

-mania = State of mental disorder, psychosis

-megaly = Enlargement, abnormal enlargement

-mnesia = Condition pertaining to memory

-noia = Condition pertaining to the mind

-oid = Resembling, to resemble

-oma = Tumor, neoplasm

-opia = Pertaining to visual condition

-oxia = Oxygen

-pathy = Disease

-penia = Deficiency

-pepsia = Digestion, to digest

-phagia = Eating, swallowing

-phasia = Speaking, to speak, speech

-phobia = Fear

-plasia = Formation, produce, development

-plasm = Cell, tissue substance

-plegia = Paralysis, stroke

-pnea = Breathing, to breath

-ptosis = Drooping, sagging

-ptysis = Spitting of matter

-rrhea = Flow, discharge

-rrhexis = Breaking, rupturing

-spasm = Spasm, twitching, involuntary contraction

-trophy = Food, nourishment

Examples include:

- **Amnesia** (loss of memory),

- Angiorrhexis (rupture of a vessel, usually a blood vessel),
- Anosteoplasia (failure of bone formation),
- Aphasia (condition characterized by partial or total inability to communicate),
- Apnoia (deranged thought),
- Cardiomegaly (abnormal enlargement of the heart),
- Cephaledema (edema of the head, swelling of the head),
- Cycloplegia (paralysis of the ciliary muscle),
- Epilepsy
- Hyperemesis (excessive vomiting),
- Hypermania (condition of extreme madness),
- Hypopepsia (impaired digestion usually caused by a pepsin deficiency), and
- Myopia (nearsightedness).

4. *Grammatical Suffixes*

Suffixes that mean 'Pertaining To'

Suffix = Meaning

-ac = pertaining to

-ad = pertaining to

-al = pertaining to

-ar = pertaining to

-ary = pertaining to

-ic = pertaining to

-ile = pertaining to

-ior = pertaining to

-ose = pertaining to

-ous = pertaining to

-tic = pertaining to

-us = pertaining to

-y = pertaining to

Suffixes that mean 'Condition', 'Treatment', or 'Specialist'

Suffix = Meaning

-esis = Condition

-ia = Condition

-ism = Condition

-iatry = Treatment

-ician = Specialist

-ist = Specialist

-osis = Condition

-y = Condition

Suffixes that mean 'Small', 'Little', or 'Minute

Suffix = Meaning

-cle = Indicating smallness, e.g. particle

-icle = Little

-ole = Indicating something small, e.g. arteriole

-ula = Small, little, minute

-ule = Small, e.g. valvule (a small valve)

Section 7: Acronyms, Eponyms, and Homonyms

In this section, we will cover medical acronyms that are the same or similar but hold entirely different meanings, some of the most common eponyms, as well as medical homonyms – these are medical terms which are pronounced the same or similarly but have an entirely different meaning.

1. *Medical Acronyms*

There are a significant amount of acronyms that are used in medical terminology, some of which are very common, whilst others are less often used. When deciphering the meaning of an acronym, context is key because acronyms are often similar or even identical.

Below is a list of common medical acronyms which are similar/identical but hold different meanings.:

AMA: Against medical advice

AMA: = American Medical Associated

CAT: Children's apperception test

CAT: Computerized axial tomography

CNS: Central nervous system

C&S: Culture and sensitivity (lab test)

COPD: Chronic obstructive pulmonary disease

COPE: Chronic obstructive pulmonary emphysema

ECT: Electroconvulsive therapy (shock therapy)

ECT: Enteric-coated tabled

ECT: Euglobulin clot test

MRI: Medical Research Institute

MRI: Medical records information

MRI: Magnetic resonance imaging

As the above highlights, context is key in order to avoid misinterpretation of an acronym!

The below are the most common abbreviations that you will encounter as a nurse or nursing student:

- a = before (ante)
- ABG = arterial blood gas
- ABT = antibiotic therapy
- ac = before meals (ante cibum)
- AD = right ear (auricula dexter)
- ADH = antidiuretic hormone
- ad lib = as desired
- ADA = American Diabetes Association
- am = before noon (ante meridian)
- AMA = against medical advice
- aq = water
- AS = left ear (auricula sinister)
- AU = both ears (auriculi utro)
- bid = twice a day
- BP = blood pressure
- BUN = blood urine nitrogen
- c = with
- cap = capsule
- CAD = coronary artery disease
- CAT = computerized axial tomography
- CBC = complete blood count
- CF = cystic fibrosis
- CHF = congestive heart failure
- CNS = central nervous system
- CO = cardiac output
- COPD = chronic obstructive pulmonary disease
- CPK = creatinine phosphokinase
- CSF = cerebrospinal fluid
- CVA = cerebrovascular accident

- CVP = central venous pressure
- EC = enteric coated
- ECG = electrocardiogram
- EEG = electroencephalogram
- elix = elixir
- ext = extract
- GFR = glomerular filtration rate
- GT = gastrostomy
- h = hour
- hct = hematocrit
- hgb = hemoglobin
- hs = bedtime (hour of sleep)
- ID = intradermal
- ICP = intracranial pressure
- IM = intramuscular
- IV = intravenous
- IVP = intravenous push
- IVPB = intravenous piggyback
- KVO = keep vein open
- MI = myocardial infarction
- NG = nasogastric
- NJ = nasojejunal (tube placement)
- NPO = nothing by mouth
- NS = normal saline
- OD = right eye (oculus dexter)
- oint = ointment
- OTC = over the counter
- OS = left eye (oculus sinister)
- OU = both eyes (oculo utro)
- p = after (post)

- pc = after meals (post cibum)
- per = by
- pm = after noon (post meridian)
- po = by mouth (per os)
- pr = per rectal
- prn = whenever necessary
- PT = prothrombin time
- PTT = partial prothrombin time
- q = every
- q1h = every 1 hour
- q2h = every 2 hours
- q3h = every 3 hours
- q4h = every 4 hours
- q6h = every 6 hours
- q8h = every 8 hours
- qd = every day
- qh = every hour
- qid = four times a day
- qod = every other day
- qs = quantity sufficient
- RBC = red blood count
- ROM = range of motion
- s = without
- sc = subcutaneous
- sl = sublingual
- sol = solution
- sq = subcutaneous
- SR = sustained release
- ss = one half
- S/S = signs and symptoms

- stat = immediately
- supp = suppository
- susp = suspension
- syr = syrup
- tab = tablet
- tid = three times a day
- TO = telephone order
- tr = tincture
- ung = ointment
- UTI = urinary tract infection
- VO = verbal order
- VS = vital signs
- WBC = white blood count
- WNL = within normal limits

2. *Eponyms*

Eponyms are words which describe a disease, drug, test, or something else that derives its name from a person. The following are among the most common eponyms that you should be aware of:

- Apgar score, named after Virginia Apgar (1909 – 1974)
- Alzheimer's disease, named after Alois Alzheimer (1864 – 1915)
- Cushing's syndrome, named after Harvey Williams Cushing (1869 – 1939)

- Down syndrome, named after John Haydon Down (1828 – 1896)
- Gleason grade, named after Donald Gleason (1828 – 1896)
- Hodgkin's disease, named after Thomas Hodgkin (1798 – 1866)
- Homan's sign, named after John Homans (1877 – 1954)
- Ligament of Treitz, named after Wenzel Treitz (1819 – 1872)
- Lyme disease, named after Old Lyme, a place in Connecticut US where the disease was first discovered in 1975
- Peyronie's disease, named after Francois de la Peyronie (1678 – 1747)
- Parkinson's disease, named after James Parkinson (1755 – 1824)

3. _Medical Homonyms_

Homonyms are words which are pronounced in the same way as another word with a different meaning. Sometimes they are even spelled the same. There are a number of homonym words in the English vocabulary. Below are the ones found in medical terminology. Again, context is key in order to avoid misinterpretation of the term. Clear and correct pronunciation and common sense are also crucial to avoid confusion.

Medical Homonym = Meaning

Ablation = Surgical removal of

Oblation = Religious offering

Access = A means of entering/approaching

Axis = Center

Afferent = Towards the center of something

Efferent = Away from the center of something

Anecdote = A funny story

Antidote = A remedy to treat poisoning

Anuresis = Retention of urine I the bladder

Enuresis = Wetting of the bed

Aural = Pertaining to the ear

Oral = Pertaining to the mouth

Callous = Insensitive and cold

Callus = A hardened are of skin

Carotid = Artery

Parotid = Gland

Cecal = Pertaining t the cecum

Fecal = Pertaining to feces

Cholic = Related to bile, an acid

Colic = Abdominal pain (severe)

Dysphagia = Difficulty swallowing or eating

Dysphasia = Difficulty speaking

Eczema = A type of dermatitis

Exemia = The loss of fluid from the blood vessels

Effusion = Escape of fluid into tissue

Infusion = To introduce fluid into the vein or tissue

Ethanol = Alcohol

Ethenyl = Vinyl

Flanges = Projecting edges or borders

Phalanges = Bones of the toes or fingers

Graft = Tissue implant form one are to another

Graph = Diagram

Humerus = A long bone (in the upper arm)

Humorous = Funny

Ileum = A portion of the colon

Ilium = A broad bone that is part of the pelvic bone

Joule = Energy

Jowl = Flesh on the jaw, lower cheek

Labial = Liplike

Labile = Unstable

Lice = Parasite

Lyse = To break

Liver = An organ of the body

Livor = Discoloration of skin after death

Loop = An oval/circular shape produced by bending

Loupe = Magnifying glass, lens

Mnemonic = Aiding or designed to aid memory

Pneumonic = Pertaining to the lungs

Nucleide = A compound of nucleic acid

Nuclide = A kind of atom or nucleus

Osteal = Bony

Ostial = Pertaining to the ostium

Palpation = Process of feeling with the fingers

Palpitation = Rapid beating of the heart

Perfusion = Pouring through or over

Profusion = Abundant

Protrusion = Extending beyond or above, jutting

Perineal = Pertaining to the genital area (perineum)

Peritoneal = Pertaining to the abdominal, pelvic cavities (peritoneum)

Peroneal = Vein (in the leg)

Plane = Anatomic (imaginary) level

Plain = Plain X-rays (radiography)

Pleuritis = Inflammation of the pleura of the lung

Pruritis = Itching

Plural = Multiple

Pleural = Pertaining to the lung =

Prostatic = Pertaining to the prostate gland

Prosthetic = An artificial device that replaces a body part

Psychosis = Mental disorder

Sycosis = Inflammation of the hair follicles

Radical = Drastic, progressive, extensive

Radicle = Smallest branch of a vessel

Scleroderma = Hardening of the skin

Scleredema = Swelling of the face

Venus = Second planet from the sun

Venous = Pertaining to the vein

Section 8: Formation of Plurals: 10 Rules

Pluralizing medical terms is different from pluralizing in everyday English language. There are 10 main rules when it comes to pluralizing medical terms which will be covered in this section.

Rule 1: Terms that end in "a": for plural add an "e".

Examples include:

- Axilla (singular) – Axillae (plural)
- Bursa (singular) – Bursae (plural
- Vertebra (singular) – Vertebrae (plural)

Rule 2: Terms that end in "um": for plural replace it with "a".

Examples include:

- Antrum (singular) – Antra (plural)
- Bacterium (singular) – Bacteria (plural)
- Labium (singular) – Labia (plural)

Rule 3: Terms that end in "us": for plural replace it with "i".

Examples include:

- Bronchus (singular) – Bronchi (plural)
- Coccus (singular) – Cocci (plural)
- Meniscus (singular) – Menisci (plural)

There are however exceptions to this rule which include the following words:

- Corpus (singular) – Corpora (plural)
- Meatus (singular) stays the same: Meatus (plural)
- Plexus (singular) – Plexuses (plural)
- Viscus (singular) – Viscera (plural)

Rule 4: Terms that end in "is": for plural change it to "es".

Examples include:

- Diagnosis (singular) – Diagnoses (plural)
- Exostosis (singular) – Exostoses (plural)
- Prognosis (singular) – Prognoses (plural)

There are again exceptions to this rule which include the following words:

- Epididymis (singular) – Epididymides (plural)
- Femur (singular) – Femora (plural)
- Iris (singular) – Irides (plural)

Rule 5: Terms that end in "ma" or "oma": for plural change to "mata".

It is important to note that for the medical terms that fall under this category, the English plural is also acceptable. Examples include:

- Carcinoma (singular) – Carcinomata (plural), Carcinomas (English plural)
- Fibroma (singular) – Fibromata (plural), Fibromas (English plural)
- Leiomyoma (singular) – Leiomyomata (plural), Leiomyomas (English Plural)

Rule 6: Terms that end in "x": for plural replace the x with "ces".

Examples include:

- Appendix (singular) – Appendices (plural)
- Calyx (singular) – Calices (plural)
- Thorax (singular) – Thoraces (plural)

An exception to this rule applies to all terms that end in 'nx'.

Rule 7: Terms that end in "nx": for plural replace it with "nges".

Examples include:

- Larynx (singular) – Larynges (plural)
- Phalanx (singular) – Phalanges (plural)

Rule 8: Terms that end in "y": for plural replace it with "ies".

Examples include:

- Bronchoscopy (singular) – Bronchoscopies (plural)
- Endoscopy (singular) – Endoscopies (plural)
- Therapy (singular) – Therapies (plural)

Rule 9: Terms that end in "itis": for plural replace it with "itides".

Examples include:

- Arthritis (singular) – Arthrides (plural)
- Meningitis (singular) – Meningitides (plural)
- Neuritis (singular) – Neuritides or Neuritises (plural)

Rule 10: Latin medical terms that consists of both a noun and an adjective: pluralize both terms

- Condyloma acuminatum (singular) – Condylomata acuminate (plural)

- Placenta previa (singular) – Placentae previae (plural)

Section 9: Medical Terms Related to Body Structure and Organization

1. *Anatomical Planes*

Anatomical planes are hypothetical planes that are used identify a specific location or area by transecting the human body into different parts.

Below are the three main planes that are used to divide the body in half, from right to left, and top from bottom.

- **The frontal or coronal plane**: This is a vertical plan that separates the front from the back of the body, i.e. the anterior form the posterior and the ventral from the dorsal.
- **The sagittal plane**: The sagittal plane, also known as lateral, is a vertical plan that separates the body into right and left sides. **The midsagittal or median plane** is a specific sagittal plane that divides the body into right and left at the body's exact midline.
- **The transverse plane:** The transverse plane, also known as horizontal or axial plane, is a horizontal plane that is runs parallel to the ground and through the waistline. It divides the body into upper and lower halves.

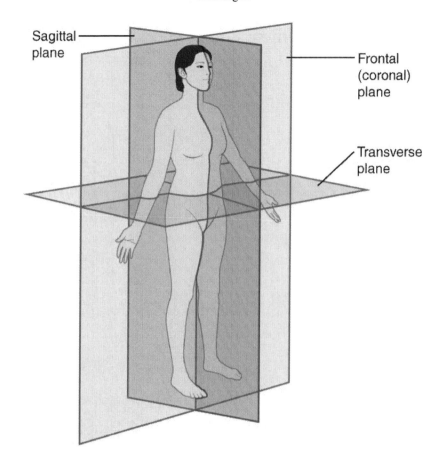

Sagittal plane

Frontal (coronal) plane

Transverse plane

2. _Body Positions_

There are certain words that are used within the medical sector to describe specific body positions.

- **Anatomical position:** This is when the body is standing erect with the arms at each side, the palms facing forward, and the feet are side by side, with parallel legs and the toes pointing forward.

- **Erect**: This is the standing position.

- **Decubitus position:** This is the posture assumed by the patient lying down, i.e. the position assumed when lying down.

- **Dorsal recumbant position:** This is the posture assumed by the patient lying on their back with the feet flat on the ground and the legs bent and separated.

- **Fowler position:** This is when the head of the patient's bed is raised about 18 inches and the body is lying on the back with the knees slightly elevated.

- **Knee-chest position:** This is the posture assumed by the patient resting on their knees, with the head and upper chest on a table and the arms cross above the head.

- **Left lateral recumbent position:** This is the posture assumed by the patient lying on their left side with the right leg (thigh and knee) drawn up.

- **Lithotomy position:** This is the posture assumed by the patient lying on their back with the legs flexed non the abdomen, thighs apart.

- **Prone:** This is the lying face down position.

- **Sims positon:** This is the posture assumed by the patient lying on their left side, with the right leg drawn up high and forward and their left arm along the back.

- **Supine position:** This is when the body is lying flat on their back with the legs straight out.

- **Trendelenburg position:** This is the posture assumed by the patient lying on their back with the head lowered by tilting the bed back at a 45-degree angle.

3. _Body Regions_

Medical terminology is also used to specifically identify a body region. In this section, we will have a look at two major areas: the abdominal area and the spinal column, as well as other important small regions of the body. It is important to be aware of these medical terms not only during practice, but also in preparation for medical and nursing examinations, and to remember that these terms were specifically designed for directional purposes. The regions of the abdomen and divisions of the spinal column are particularly prone to come up in examinations.

THE ABDOMINAL AREA

The abdominal area is divided into nine anatomic regions, the division of which facilitates the diagnosis of abdominal problems.

The portion in the center is the **umbilical region**. This is the area that surrounds the umbilicus (navel). The organs that are found in the umbilical region include the Umbilicus, Jejunum, Ileum, and the Duodenum. On either side of the umbilical region are the right and left lumbar regions. The **right lumber region** comprises of the Gallbladder, the Liver, and the Right Colon. The left lumber region comprises of the Descending Colon and the Left Kidney.

The region directly above the umbilical region is called the **epigastric region.** The organs that are found in this region include the Stomach, Liver, Pancreas, Duodenum, Spleen, and the Adrenal Glands. To the right and left of the epigastric region are the right and left hypochondriac regions. The **right hypochondriac region** comprises of the Liver, Gallbladder, Right Kidney, and the Small Intestine.

The **left hypochondriac region** comprises of the Spleen, Colon, Left Kidney, and the Pancreas.

The region directly below the umbilical region is called the **hypogastric region**, which is the region of the abdomen below the navel. The organs that are found in the hypogastric region include the following: Urinary Bladder, Sigmoid Colon, and the Female Reproductive Organs. To the right and left of the hypogastric region are the right and left iliac regions. The **right iliac region (or fossa)** comprises of the Appendix and the Cecum. The **left iliac region (fossa)** comprises of the Descending Colon and the Sigmoid Colon.

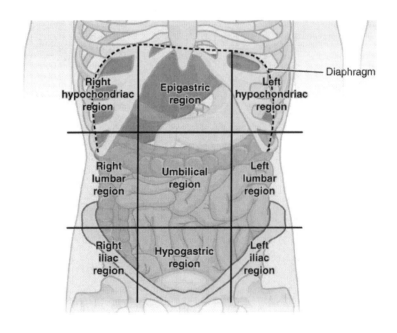

When a patient is being examined, clinical regions are used

to divide the abdominal area into four equal quadrants.

- **The right upper quadrant (RUQ)**: This region is often assessed to localize pain as well as tenderness. This region is often tender in clients with cholecystitis, hepatitis, or a developing peptic ulcer. Important organs that are found in this quadrant include the liver, the gall bladder, and parts of the small and large intestines.

- **The left upper quadrant (LUQ):** This region is often tender in clients with abnormalities of the intestines and in clients with appendicitis. Important organs that are found in this quadrant include the stomach, pancreas, spleen, the left portion of the liver, and parts of the small and large intestines.

- **The right lower quadrant (RLQ)**: This region, which stretches from the median plane to the right side of the body and from the umbilical plane to the right inguinal ligament, is often tender and painful in clients with appendicitis. Important organs that are found in this quadrant include the appendix, the upper portion of the colon, the right ovary, the right ureter, the Fallopian tube, and parts of the small and large intestines.

- **The left lower quadrant (LLQ):** This region, which is located below the umbilicus plane, is usually tender and painful in clients with ovarian cysts or a pelvic inflammation. Abdominal pain in this region can also be a symptom of colitis, diverticulitis, or ureteral colic. Tumors in the LLQ can be indicative of colon or ovarian cancer. Important organs found in this region include the left ovary, the left ureter, the Fallopian tube, and parts of the small and large intestine.

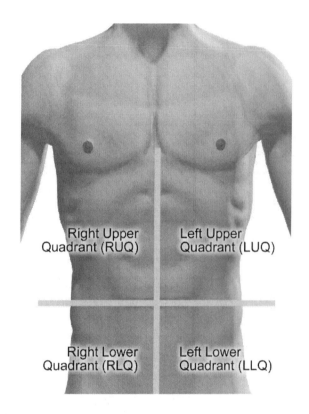

THE SPINAL COLUMN

The spinal column is divided into five regions:

- **The cervical region (abbreviation C)** consists of seven cervical vertebrae, C1 to C7, which are the smallest of the true vertebrae. They are located in the neck region closest to the skill.

- **The thoracic or dorsal region (abbreviation T or D)** consists of 12 thoracic or dorsal vertebrae: T1 to T12 or D1 to D12. They are located in the chest region of the spine.

- **The lumbar region (abbreviation L),** sometimes referred to as the lower spine, consists of five lumbar vertebrae, L1 to L5. The lumbar region is found at the flank or loin area between the ribs and the hip bone.

- **The sacral region (abbreviation S),** consists of five bones, S1 to S5, which are located at the bottom of the spine. These five bones are fused together to form one bone: **the sacrum.**

- **The coccygeal region,** also referred to as the tailbone, is a small bone at the very bottom of the spine. It is composed of four vertebrae that are fused together to form one bone: **the coccyx.**

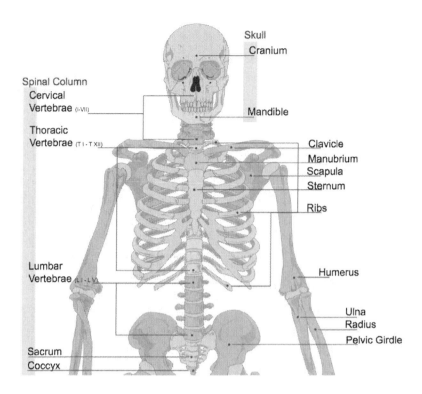

SMALL REGIONS OF THE BODY

- **Auricular region:** This is the region around the ears
- **Axillary:** The armpit region
- **Clavicular:** The region on either side of two slender bones
- **Infraorbital:** The region below the eyes
- **Infrascapular:** This is the region on each side of the chest, down to the last rib
- **Inguinal:** The region of the groin, i.e. the depressed area of the abdominal wall near the thigh

- **Interscapular:** This is the region on the back between the shoulder blades (the scapulae)
- **Lumbar:** The region of the lower back between the ribs and the pelvis below the infrascapular area
- **Mammary:** The breast area
- **Mental:** The chin area
- **Occipital:** The lower posterior region of the head
- **Orbital:** The region around the eyes
- **Pectoral:** The chest area
- **Perineal:** The region between the anus and the external reproductive organs (the perineum)
- **Popliteal:** The area behind the knee
- **Pubic:** The area above the pubis and below the hypogastric region
- **Sacral:** The area above the sacrum, between the hipbones
- **Sternal:** The area over the sternum
- **Submental:** The area below the chin
- **Supraclavicular:** The area above the clavicles

4. _Body Cavities_

The body is not a solid structure but is rather composed of cavities (fluid-filled spaces) which contain body organs.

The Dorsal Body Cavity, located on the back part of the body, comprises of:

- **The Cranial Cavity**, which is enclosed by the skull and contains the brain.
- **The Spinal Cavity,** which contains the spinal cord.

The Ventral Body Cavity, located on the front of the body, comprises of:

- **The Thoracic or Chest Cavity:** This cavity contains the esophagus, lungs, trachea, heart, and aorta.
- **The Abdominopelvic Cavity**, which comprises of:
  - o **The Abdominal Cavity:** This cavity contains the stomach, intestines, liver, spleen, gallbladder, pancreases, ureters, and kidneys.
  - o **The Pelvic Cavity:** This cavity contains the urinary bladder, urethra, rectum, uterus, part of the large intestine, and the reproductive organs.

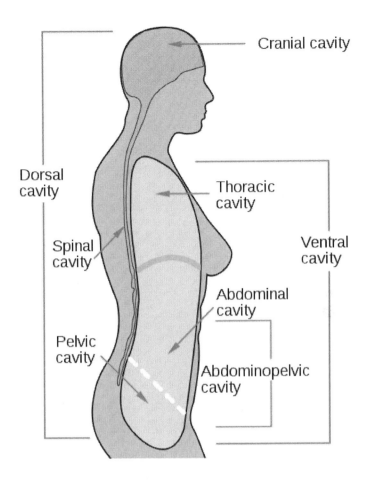

5. *Body Parts*

Below are medical terms which are frequently used in the medical or clinical setting when referring to some common body. Familiarity with these terms is therefore crucial.

- **Acromial:** Point of the shoulder
- **Antebrachial:** Forearm

- **Axillary:** Armpit
- **Brachial:** Arm
- **Buccal:** Cheek
- **Carpal:** Wrist
- **Celiac:** Abdomen
- **Cephalic:** Head
- **Cervical:** Neck
- **Costal:** Ribs
- **Coxal:** Hip
- **Crural:** Leg
- **Cubital:** Elbow
- **Digital:** Finger
- **Dorsum:** Back
- **Femoral:** Thigh
- **Frontal:** Forehead
- **Genital:** Reproductive organs
- **Gluteal:** Buttocks
- **Mental:** Chin
- **Nasal:** Nose
- **Oral:** Mouth
- **Otic:** Ear
- **Palmar:** Palm of the hand
- **Patellar:** Kneecap or kneepan
- **Pedal:** Foot
- **Pelvic:** Pelvis
- **Plantar:** Sole of the foot
- **Tarsal:** Tarsus of the foot, instep of the foot
- **Umbilical:** Navel
- **Vertebral:** Spinal column

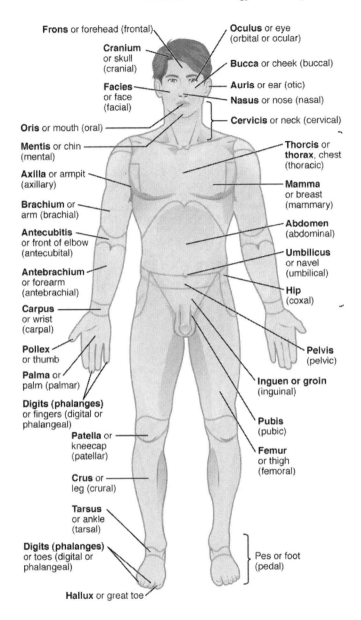

Frons or forehead (frontal)

Cranium or skull (cranial)

Facies or face (facial)

Oris or mouth (oral)

Mentis or chin (mental)

Axilla or armpit (axillary)

Brachium or arm (brachial)

Antecubitis or front of elbow (antecubital)

Antebrachium or forearm (antebrachial)

Carpus or wrist (carpal)

Pollex or thumb

Palma or palm (palmar)

Digits (phalanges) or fingers (digital or phalangeal)

Patella or kneecap (patellar)

Crus or leg (crural)

Tarsus or ankle (tarsal)

Digits (phalanges) or toes (digital or phalangeal)

Hallux or great toe

Oculus or eye (orbital or ocular)

Bucca or cheek (buccal)

Auris or ear (otic)

Nasus or nose (nasal)

Cervicis or neck (cervical)

Thorcis or **thorax**, chest (thoracic)

Mamma or breast (mammary)

Abdomen (abdominal)

Umbilicus or navel (umbilical)

Hip (coxal)

Pelvis (pelvic)

Inguen or groin (inguinal)

Pubis (pubic)

Femur or thigh (femoral)

Pes or foot (pedal)

Section 10: Medical Terms of Body Systems

In the previous section, we discussed the organization of the body and the relative terminology that is applied to refer to them. This section builds on your pre-existing knowledge and understanding of medical terminology. You will already be familiar with a lot of the combining forms and root words mentioned in this section. Instead, this section is designed to help you categorize all the terms that you have learned and to apply them accurately to the body system that you are working with. We will cover all the main combining forms that relate to a specific body system, some specific prefixes and suffixes, their respective definitions, as well as provide common examples.

1. *The Cardiovascular System*

Combining Form = Meaning

Aden(o) = Gland

Angi(o), Vas(o) = Vessel

Aort(o) = Aorta

Arteri(o) = Artery

Ather(o) = Fatty plaque

Atri(o) = Atrium

Cardi(o) = Heart

Erythr(o) = Red

Hem(o), Hemat(o) = Blood

Leuc(o), Leuk(o) = White

Lymph(o) = Lymph

Phleb(o), Ven(o) = Vein

Splen(o) = Spleen

Thromb(o) = Clot

Ventricul(o) = Ventricle

Examples include:

- **Angio**plasty (surgical repair of the blood vessel),
- **Athero**sclerosis (disease of the arteries characterized by the deposits of fatty plaques),
- **Erythro**cytes (red blood cells),
- **Leuko**cytes (white blood cells),
- **Lympho**ma (tumor that is found in the lymph), and
- **Splen**ectomy (surgical removal of the spleen).

2. *The Respiratory System*

Combining Form/Suffix = Meaning

Aer(o) = Air

Atel(o) = Imperfect

Bronch(o/io) = Bronchus

Bronchiol(o) = Bronchioles

Laryng(o) = Larynx

Lob(o) = Lobes

Muc(o) = Mucus

Nas(o), Rhin(o) = Nose

Ox(o) = Oxygen

Pharyng(o) = Pharynx

Pleur(o) = Pleura

Pneum(o), Pnemon(o) = Lung, air

Pulmon(o) = Lung

-ptysis = Spitting, to spit

Sinus(o) = Sinus(es)

Spir(o) = Breathing, to breath

Tonsill(o) = Tonsil(s)

Trache(o) = Trachea, windpipe

Examples include:

- **Bronchiol**itis (inflammation of the bronchi),
- **Laryng**ectomy (surgical removal of the larynx),
- Hemo**ptysis** (condition of spitting up blood),
- Hyp**oxia** (the condition of deficient, below normal levels of oxygen),
- **Pleur**isy (inflammation of the pleura),
- **Pneumo**nitis or **Pneumo**nia (inflammation of a lung), and
- **Spiro**meter (device used to measure the amount of air a patient inhales and exhales).

3. _The Gastrointestinal System_

Combining Form/Suffix = Meaning

Abdomin(o) = Abdomen

Aden(o) = Gland

Aliment(o) = Food, nourishment

Amyl(o) = Starch

An(o) = Anus

Append(o), Appendic(o) = Appendix

-ase = Enzyme

Bucc(o) = Cheek

Cec(o) = Cecum

Cheil(o) = Lips

Cholecyst(o) = Gallbladder

Choled(o) = Common bile duct

Col(o), Colon(o) = Colon

Dent(i/o), Odont(o) = Tooth, teeth

Duoden(o) = Duodenum

Enter(o) = Small intestine

Epiglott(o) = Epiglottis

Esophag(o) = Esophagus

Gastr(o) = Stomach

Gloss(o), Lingu(o) = Tongue

Hepat(o) = Liver

Ile(o) = Ileum

Intestin(o) = Intestine

Jejun(o) = Jejunum

Lith(o) = Stone, calculus

Or(o), Stomat(o) = Mouth

Pancreat(o) = Pancreas

Periton(o) = Peritoneum

Pharyng(o) = Pharynx

Proct(o), Rect(o) = Rectum

Sial(o) = Saliva

Sigmoid(o) = Sigmoid colon

Examples include:

- **Amylase** (enzyme that breaks down starch),
- Ankylo**gloss**ia (the condition of being tongue tied),
- **Cholecysto**lithiasis (the condition of having gallstones),
- **Colo**stomy (artificial/surgical opening into the colon),
- **Gastrointestin**al (pertaining to the stomach and the liver),
- **Hepat**itis (inflammation of the liver),
- **Oropharyng**eal (pertaining to the mouth and the throat),
- **Sialaden**itis (inflammation of the salivary glands),
- **Siallith**ectomy (surgical removal of the salivary stones), and
- **Sigmoid**ectomy (surgical removal of the sigmoid colon).

4. *The Endocrine System*

Combining Form/Suffix = Meaning

Gluc(o), Glyc(o) = Sugar, sweet

-oid = Resembling

-ose = Sugar

Parathyroid(o) = Parathyroid glands

Thym(o) = Thymus gland

Thyr(o) = Thyroid gland, shield

Toxic(o) = Toxin, posin

Examples include:

- **Gluco**suria or **Glyco**suria (the presence of sugar in the urine),
- Sucr**ose,** Lact**ose,** Gluc**ose** (different types of sugars),
- **Thymo**sin (a hormone excreted by the thymus gland),
- Thy**roid** (literally means resembling a shield), and
- **Thyrotoxico**sis (condition of the thyroid being poisoned).

5. *The Integumentary System*

Combining Form = Meaning

Adip(o), Lip(o) = Fat

Albin(o), Leuk(o) = White, without color

Cutane(o), Derm(o) = Skin

Dermat(o), Integument(o) = Skin

Cyan(o) = Blue

Erythem(o) = Red

Melan(o) = Black

Onych(o) = Nail

Scler(o) = Hard, hardenining

Xanth(o), Icter(o) = Yellow

Xer(o) = Dry

Examples include:

- **Adipo**se tissue (the layer just below the skin which consists mostly of fat cells),
- **Icter**ic (displaying a yellow discoloration of the skin),
- **Leukoderma** (the condition of abnormal patches of white skin),
- **Lipo**ma (a fatty benign tumor),
- **Onycho**mycosis (fungal infection of the nails), and
- **Scleroderma** (the condition of hardened skin).

6. _The Musculoskeletal System_

Combining Form = Meaning

Ankylos(o) = Stiffening

Arthr(o) = Joint

Carp(o) = Wrist (bones)

Cervic(o) = Neck

Chondr(o) = Cartilage

Cost(o) = Ribs

Crani(o) = Skull

Dactyl(o) = Digit

Femor(o) = Femur, thighbone

Fibul(o) = Fibula (smaller bone in the calf)

Humer(o) = Humerus (upper bone in the arm)

Ili(o) = Ilium (pelvic bone)

Lamin(o) = Lamina of a vertebra

Mandibul(o) = Mandible (the lower jaw)

Maxill(o) = Maxilla (the upper jaw)

Muscul(o), My(o) = Muscle

Orth(o) = Straight, straighten

Oste(o) = Bone

Patell(o) = Patella, kneecap

Pelv(i) = Pelvis

Phalang(o) = Fingers or toes

Rachi(o), Spondyl(o) = Vertebra(e), spine
Vertebr(o) = Vertebra(e), spine

Stern(o) = Sternum, breastbone

Ten(o), Tend(o), Tendin(o) = Tendon

Tibi(o) = Tibia, shin

Examples include:

- **Ankylos**ing **spondyl**itis (the abnormal stiffening of the spine),
- **Costo**chondritis (inflammation of the cartilage around the ribs),
- **Femor**al artery (an artery which is found near the thighbone),
- **Lamin**ectomy (the surgical removal of a portion of the vertebrae),
- **Rachi**tis, **Spondyl**itis (inflammation of the vertebrae or the spine), and
- Sub**sternal** pain (pain that is found just below the breastbone).

7. *The Sensory System*

Root word, Prefix, Suffix = Meaning

Audi(o) = Sound, hearing

Aur(o), Ot(o) = Ear

Blephar(o) = Eyelid

Conjunctiv(o) = Conjunctiva(e)

Corne(o) = Cornea

-cusis (suffix) = To hear, hearing

Myring(o), Tympan(o) = Eardrum

Ocul(o), Ophthalm(o) = Eye

Olfact(o) = Smell

Presby- (prefix) = Aging, elderly

-ptosis = (suffix) = Sagging, drooping

Retin(o) = Retina

Exaples include:

- **Blepharoptosis** (the condition of having a sagging eyelid),
- **Corne**al (pertaining to the cornea of the eye),
- Micr**oti**a (the condition of having very small ears),
- **Ophthalmo**logist (specialist in eye diseases and treatment), and

- **Presbycusis** (the condition of diminished hearing associated with aging).

8. *The Nervous System*

Combining Form = Meaning

Cerebell(o) = Cerebellum

Electr(o) = Electricity

Encephal(o), Cerebr(o) = Brain, cerebrum

Mening(o) = Meninges

Neur(o) = Nerve

Phas(o) = Speech

Examples include:
- **Aphas**ia (condition of being unable to speak, e.g. in patients who have suffered a stoke),
- **Meningo**coccal (infection of the meninges),
- **Neur**algia (pain in a nerve), and
- Viral **encephal**itis (inflammation of the brain by a virus).

9. *The Urinary System*

Combining Form = Meaning

Bacteri(o) = Bacteria

Cyst(o) = Bladder, sac

Glomerul(o) = Glomerulus

Hemat(o) = Blood

Lith(o) = Stone, calculus

Nephr(o), Ren(o) = Nephron

Noct(o) = Night

Py(o) = Pus

Pyel(o) = Renal pelvis

Ur(o), Urin(o) = Urine

Ureter(o) = Ureter

Urethr(o) = Urethra

Examples include:

- **Bacteriur**ia (presence of bacteria in the urine),
- **Nephro**lithiasis (the condition of having kidney stones),
- **Noct**uria (condition of having to wake and pass urine at night),

- **Pyelolitho**tomy (the surgical removal of kidney stones from the renal pelvis),
- **Py**uria (the presence of pus in the urine), and
- **Urino**meter (device used to measure the specific gravity of urine).

10. *The Reproductive System*

Combining Form = Meaning

Amni(o) = Amnion

Cervic(o) = Cervix of the uterus, neck

Colp(o), Vagin(o) = Vagina

Embry(o) = Embryo

Gravida = Pregnancy

Gyn(o), Gynec(o) = Female

Hyster(o), Metr(o), Uter(o) = Uterus

Lact(o) = Milk

Mamm(o), Mast(o) = Breast

Men(o) = Menstruation

Nat(o) = Birth

Oophor(o), Ovari(o) = Ovary

Orch(o/i/io/d/do), Test(o) = Testes

Ov(o) = Egg

Salping(o) = Fallopian tube

Sperm(o), Spermat(o) = Sperm

Examples include:

- **Colpo**scopy (visual examination of the vagina)
- **Meno**pause (marks the period of time when a woman ceases to have monthly periods)
- Ne**onat**e (a newborn)
- Nulli **gravida** (term that says that a woman is pregnant)
- **Oophor**ectomy (surgical removal of an ovary)
- **Ov**al (shaped like an egg)
- **Salping**itis (inflammation of the Fallopian tube)
- **Vagin**itis (inflammation of the vagina).

Section 11: Final Notes

I would like to take this opportunity to thank you for purchasing this book. I hope you now have a solid foundation, and that this guide has helped you equip yourself with the knowledge you need to understand, deconstruct, and build medical terminology.

My final piece of advice - no matter how diligent you are in your studies, your best learning will come from proactively deconstructing medical terms and understanding the architecture and origin of a term, as well as to constantly refresh and build on your knowledge as you progress.

I sincerely wish you the best of luck in your nursing career.

Best wishes,

Eva Regan

Made in the USA
Lexington, KY
27 February 2017